The Pink Salt Trick Recipes for Weight Loss

21-Day Natural Hormone Reset to Feel Lighter, Calmer, and Stronger with Salt Rituals That Support Hormonal Balance, Cravings, and Metabolic Health

Abigail Douglas

1

Table of Contents

3

Disclaimer

This book is intended for informational purposes only and does not constitute medical advice. Always consult with a qualified healthcare provider before beginning any new health, nutrition, or wellness program. The author and publisher disclaim any liability for any adverse effects resulting from the use or application of the information contained herein.

Preface

Are you tired of dieting and still gaining weight? Struggling with belly fat, cravings, or fatigue that no workout or meal plan seems to fix?

You're not broken. You're just missing the natural weight loss ritual your body was designed for — and it starts with something as simple as pink salt.

Introducing *The Pink Salt Trick Recipes for Weight Loss* — a groundbreaking, holistic wellness guide created especially for women over 40 who are ready to stop the cycle of restriction, shame, and metabolic confusion.

This isn't a diet. It's a 21-day hormone reset plan that uses pink salt for weight loss, bloat relief, adrenal recovery, and mood support — all without extreme workouts or complicated regimens.

If you've ever asked, "Why can't I lose belly fat over 40?", you're not alone. The truth is, many women experience adrenal fatigue weight gain, mineral imbalance and cravings, and cortisol belly fat spikes during perimenopause and beyond. This book offers a no-diet weight loss plan that works with your hormones — not against them.

Inside, you'll discover:

- The salt water flush for bloating that gently resets your gut and digestive system
- A full 21-day hormone reset calendar tailored to your energy, mood, and menstrual cycle
- Rituals to stop sugar cravings naturally and restore adrenal-thyroid-cortisol balance
- Quick recipes like the easy morning ritual to lose weight and night-time salt infusions that promote sleep and fat-burning
- A flexible, anti-inflammatory weight loss guide that also acts as a natural remedy for PMS bloating and menopausal discomfort

- Strategic salt pairings that target everything from water retention to cravings, including natural energy boosts for women

- How to use pink salt detox for belly fat alongside herbs, adaptogens, and functional foods

- A sustainable, gentle detox that actually works — no pills, powders, or food group eliminations

- Practical advice on how to reset hormones without pills while supporting your thyroid for weight loss

This book was written for women asking bigger questions:

- "How can I feel lighter without starving?"

- "What's a fat-burning ritual without dieting that won't disrupt my day?"

- "How do I balance my hormones naturally and feel calm in my own skin?"

Whether you're navigating perimenopause weight gain, struggling to stop sugar cravings naturally, or just looking for a belly bloat remedy for women that doesn't involve another cleanse — this book gives you the tools to reclaim your metabolism with rhythm, not restriction.

With a unique blend of natural weight loss rituals, salt-based healing recipes, and mindset shifts, *The Pink Salt Trick* is more than a wellness guide — it's a roadmap to becoming the most calm, light, and energized version of yourself.

It's time to nourish, not deprive. To reset, not restrict.

Because when your minerals are balanced, your hormones follow — and weight loss becomes the side effect of healing, not the goal.

Introduction

"Why This Book Works When Diets Don't"

If you've tried everything—counting calories, cutting carbs, fasting until your hands shake, or working out like it's your second job—only to feel more exhausted, bloated, and stuck in a body that doesn't reflect your efforts... you are not alone. You are not failing. The system is.

Most weight loss advice given to women is built on one core message: restrict more. Eat less, deny more, push harder. But what if the problem isn't your willpower? What if your body isn't broken—but burned out? What if the path to fat loss, bloat relief, and hormonal balance isn't another punishing plan... but a mineral you've been taught to fear?

That mineral is salt.

More specifically: Himalayan pink salt, one of the most misunderstood and underutilized natural tools for women's metabolism, digestion, energy, and hormone balance.

Why Women Struggle with Dieting and Hormonal Fat

Unlike men, a woman's body is not designed to run on willpower and rigid discipline. It's designed to respond to rhythm—to cycles, hydration, minerals, sleep, and subtle stress cues. When you throw your system into survival mode through restriction, the hormonal consequences can be devastating. Your cortisol spikes, your thyroid slows, and your metabolism goes into hibernation. And yet, the weight doesn't move. The cravings intensify. The bloat becomes permanent. The energy crashes. You try again—and it gets worse.

This isn't just frustrating. It's physiological.

Hormonal weight gain—especially around the belly—isn't just about fat. It's about imbalance. It's about chronic inflammation, poor digestion, sluggish adrenals, underfed thyroids, and mineral depletion. And pink salt, believe it or not, holds the key to all of these.

Why Pink Salt is a Metabolic Ally—Not the Enemy

Pink Himalayan salt is rich in over 80 trace minerals, including magnesium, potassium, and iodine in natural ratios your body recognizes. Unlike chemically stripped table salt, pink salt is electrically alive—it supports cellular hydration, balances electrolytes, and nourishes the glands that regulate metabolism and energy.

For women dealing with fatigue, stubborn weight, water retention, or mood swings, pink salt isn't just seasoning—it's medicine.

This book shows you how to use it that way.

You won't need to starve yourself. You won't need to track points or macros or steps. You'll learn how to wake up and replenish your body, not punish it. You'll drink simple, delicious tonics that trigger fat-burning, ease digestion, reduce cravings, calm your nervous system, and reintroduce you to a body that actually listens.

And it starts with a tiny pinch of pink salt.

The Gut–Adrenal–Thyroid Connection, Explained Simply

At the center of your energy, mood, and weight is a delicate triangle of systems:

- Your gut, where digestion, absorption, and immune function begin.
- Your adrenals, which govern stress response and blood sugar.
- Your thyroid, which drives metabolism, warmth, and hormonal rhythm.

When one of these breaks down, the others follow. Dieting can wreck all three. Pink salt helps repair them—by increasing stomach acid for digestion, hydrating cells to reduce adrenal strain, and delivering essential minerals to help your thyroid produce hormones efficiently.

We're not talking magic. We're talking biological restoration.

The morning salt water ritual you'll learn in this book is backed by a century of hydrotherapy and modern functional nutrition. The recipes are based on simple food chemistry and real hormonal needs. The 21-day plan is structured not to restrict you—but to bring your body back online, one small shift at a time.

Who This Book is For

This book is for the woman who's tired of extremes.

It's for the woman who's tried keto, paleo, vegan, Whole30, IF, and detox teas—and ended up more confused and inflamed than before.

It's for the woman who wakes up bloated, drags through her mornings, can't focus by 2pm, and punishes herself with guilt when her pants feel tight.

It's for the woman who wants her life back—not just a smaller dress size.

If that's you, welcome.

You won't find guilt here. You won't find shame or complicated charts or metabolic jargon. What you will find is a return to simplicity—to nourishment, balance, energy, and trust in your body again.

You'll find yourself sipping warm lemon salt water at sunrise, watching your belly flatten, your energy rise, and your skin glow.

You'll learn to listen—to what your body needs, not what the diet industry shouts.

You'll realize it's not about eating less. It's about giving more of what your body actually craves.

And you'll see—day by day, ritual by ritual—that the lightness you've been chasing doesn't come from less food... it comes from less inflammation, less imbalance, and less stress.

What You'll Gain From This Book

By the end of this journey, you'll know how to:

- **Debloat fast and naturally** with mineral-based recipes

- **Burn fat without dieting**, using daily salt rituals

- **Balance your hormones**, especially if you struggle with PMS, thyroid issues, or menopause

- **Sustain clean energy** throughout the day—without caffeine or crashes

- **Heal your gut and digestion**, improving everything from mood to metabolism

- **Reclaim your calm and confidence** without punishing your body to earn it

You won't just lose weight.

You'll lose the belief that weight loss has to be a war against your own biology.

So go ahead. Flip the page. Pick up a spoon. Your reset starts now— with something you've had all along.

A pinch of pink salt.

Chapter 1

The Pink Salt Trick — What It Is & Why It Works

It started with a morning ritual so simple, it almost felt too gentle to be effective.

A spoonful of warm lemon water, a pinch of pink salt, and a quiet moment before the day began.

But within a week, something changed. Less bloating. Less brain fog. Cravings faded. Clothes fit looser. Energy returned—slowly, but unmistakably. And for the first time in a long time, weight began to shift—not from punishment, but from alignment.

That's the Pink Salt Trick.

Not a gimmick. Not a detox scam. Not another short-term fix pretending to be sustainable. The Pink Salt Trick is about nourishing your metabolism, hormones, and digestion from the inside out—by returning to something your body has been silently begging for:

- Real minerals.

- And in a world addicted to extremes, this trick is a return to truth.

The Story Behind the Pink Salt Trick

Let's be honest: when most of us hear the word "salt," we think of something to fear. We're told to avoid it, restrict it, or find a low-sodium version of whatever we're eating. Salt has been blamed for everything from high blood pressure to water retention to belly bloat. So we follow the advice. We cut it down, drink more water, eat bland food—and wonder why we're still tired, still swollen, still stuck.

But here's what they don't tell you: it's not salt that's the problem.

It's the wrong kind of salt—and the absence of the right kind.

31

Table salt—the bleached, refined, stripped-down version found in processed food—is not what your body was designed to use. It's missing the very minerals that give salt its life-supporting properties. It's been chemically altered, often with additives and anti-caking agents that serve shelf stability, not health.

In contrast, *Himalayan pink salt* is what salt was meant to be: whole, unrefined, naturally structured to deliver trace minerals your cells actually recognize. It contains over 80 bioavailable minerals, including magnesium, potassium, calcium, and iron—each one supporting a vital function in your metabolism, hydration, hormonal rhythm, or nervous system.

That's where the trick begins.

By adding a small, intentional amount of this mineral-rich salt to your morning routine, you're not "salting your way to weight gain"—you're restoring the foundation of your body's metabolic engine. And that one small shift begins to ripple outward in profound ways.

Why Mineral-Rich Salt Changes Everything

Let's break it down simply.

Your body runs on electricity.

Every thought, every heartbeat, every movement is an electrical impulse that depends on minerals to flow. These minerals—called electrolytes—help transmit messages between cells, keep muscles contracting, move nutrients through membranes, and maintain your internal pH.

When you're mineral-deficient (which nearly everyone is, especially women), your body struggles to:

- Stay hydrated at the cellular level

- Digest food properly

- Produce adequate stomach acid

- Balance blood sugar

- Regulate cortisol and thyroid hormones

- Burn fat efficiently

This isn't abstract science. It's everyday fatigue. It's the 3PM crash. It's the bloat after a light meal. It's the stubborn weight that won't move, no matter how clean you eat.

Mineral-rich pink salt is like an on-switch for these systems.

It helps you absorb water instead of retaining it. It stimulates bile production, which is crucial for fat digestion. It supports adrenal health, which in turn reduces belly fat linked to stress. It balances fluid retention, eases cramps, and reduces PMS flare-ups. It even curbs sugar cravings, because your body isn't mistaking mineral deficiency for hunger.

And it doesn't take a lot. Just the right type, in the right way, at the right time.

How Salt Supports Hydration, Bile Flow,

Metabolism & Adrenal Repair

You've likely been told to "just drink more water" to lose weight or clear up your skin.

But here's the truth: water without minerals doesn't hydrate—it can actually dehydrate.

Your cells need electrolytes like sodium, magnesium, and potassium to pull water inside. Without them, the water you drink passes through your body quickly, diluting your minerals further, making you pee more, and leaving you just as thirsty, bloated, or foggy as before.

That's why adding a pinch of pink salt to your water first thing in the morning can be a game changer.

But it goes deeper.

When pink salt reaches your stomach, it stimulates hydrochloric acid production, which is essential for breaking down protein and absorbing nutrients. Poor stomach acid is a hidden cause of bloating, reflux, and food sensitivities—and it's common in stressed-out, diet-fatigued women.

Pink salt also triggers bile flow from the liver and gallbladder. Without good bile flow, fat digestion stalls, toxins build up, and hormone clearance slows down. That leads to bloating, estrogen dominance, fatigue, and—yes—stubborn fat storage.

Now pair all of that with adrenal support.

Your adrenal glands, which sit above your kidneys, regulate stress hormones like cortisol and aldosterone. These hormones affect everything from belly fat to mood to water retention. When you're chronically stressed or dieting, your adrenals get depleted—and so does your body's salt balance.

That's why salt cravings often intensify during burnout. Your body isn't sabotaging you. It's asking to be replenished.

The Truth About Bloating—and Why Salt Isn't the Enemy

Let's dismantle one of the biggest myths that keeps women inflamed and confused: the idea that salt causes bloating.

It's not salt—it's sodium in isolation, combined with dehydration, processed foods, and a lack of minerals.

When you eat processed table salt (like what's in chips, canned soup, or fast food), your body holds on to water in an attempt to dilute the harsh sodium load. You puff up. Your rings don't fit. Your belly swells.

But when you consume natural, mineral-rich pink salt, the opposite happens. Your body uses the salt to move water into the cells—

improving circulation, reducing fluid retention, and flushing out toxins more efficiently. You urinate more effectively, not excessively. You feel lighter, not swollen.

It's not about cutting out salt—it's about upgrading it.

And when you do, your digestive system responds. Your skin clears. Your energy returns. Your cycle becomes more stable. And that uncomfortable, hard-to-describe sense of inflammation begins to ease.

Daily Salt Intake: Myths, Truth, and Balance

So how much pink salt should you consume?

This is where balance matters. We're not suggesting you start salting every bite of food or drinking brine by the cup. The Pink Salt Trick is about intentional use—not overuse.

For most women, a good starting ritual is:

- ½ teaspoon of pink Himalayan salt in warm lemon water each morning

- Plus a few pinches added to whole foods throughout the day (especially if sweating or under stress)

This amount supports electrolyte balance without overloading sodium. And when paired with real food, good hydration, and rest, it becomes a daily metabolic reset.

More isn't better. Precision is.

Listen to your body. Some days you'll need more salt—after a workout, during PMS, or in the heat. Other days, you may feel balanced with less. The goal is not to "hit a number." The goal is to nourish your systems, gently and consistently.

The Foundation Has Been Laid

This chapter is the cornerstone of what you'll build on next.

Now that you understand why pink salt is not just safe—but essential—you're ready to learn how to turn it into a ritual. In the next chapter, we'll dive into the exact Daily Salt Blueprint that's helped thousands of women burn fat, ease bloat, reset cravings, and reclaim their sense of calm.

You won't need to track anything.

You'll just need to trust that sometimes, the most powerful solutions are the ones the body recognizes immediately—and pink salt is one of them.

THE PINK SALT TRICK

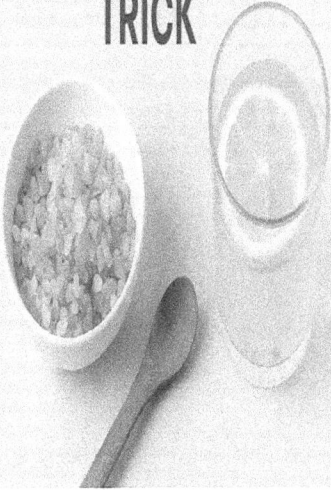

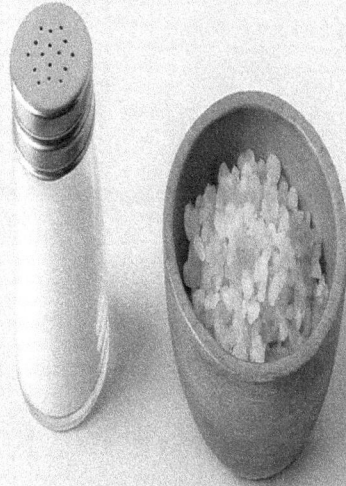

Table salt vs. pink salt

Supports hydration

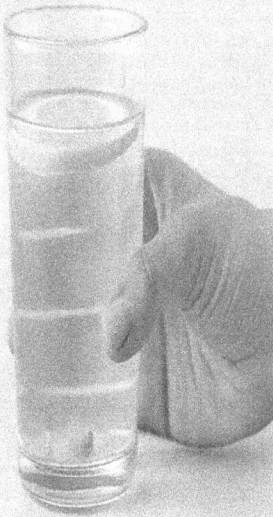

Helps metabolism

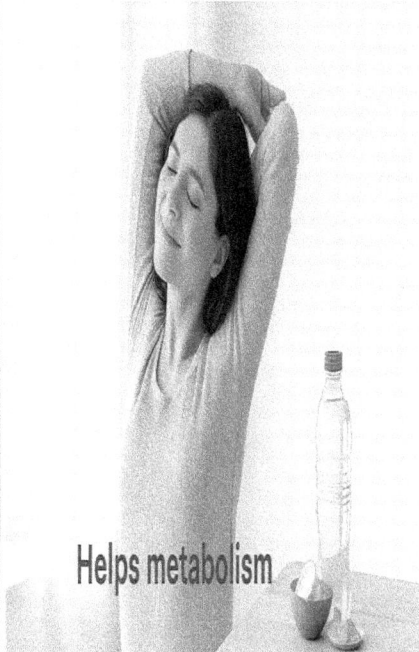

41

Chapter 2

The Daily Ritual Blueprint — Reset, Rehydrate, Reignite

You don't need more rules. You need rhythm.

If Chapter 1 helped you understand *why* pink salt works on a biological level, this chapter is where the shift begins. Because understanding isn't enough—you need a practice. Something real. Something you can do tomorrow morning that won't require weighing your food or tracking anything but your own sense of aliveness.

This is your new approach to weight loss, energy, and hormone balance—rooted not in willpower, but in ritual.

This is The Daily Salt Blueprint.

It begins in the quiet of the morning and carries you gently into the night. It's not restrictive. It's restorative. Each step is designed to give your body exactly what it needs, exactly when it needs it—based on the wisdom of your circadian rhythm, your mineral needs, and your hormonal cycles.

This is not about discipline. It's about cooperation with your biology. And it starts with salt.

The Morning Salt Water Ritual: Your Metabolism's Wake-Up Call

Before the coffee. Before the scroll. Before the stress of the day floods in.

There's a moment in the morning when your body is at a crossroads. Your system is waking up, cortisol is rising, digestion is restarting, and your metabolism is about to decide whether to burn or conserve.

43

What you do in this window matters.

The Morning Salt Water Ritual is a powerful yet gentle metabolic command. It's your way of saying to your cells, *"We're safe. You're supported. Let's burn clean, let's move energy, let's reset."*

✦ How to Prepare the Ritual

- 1 full glass (10–12 oz) of warm, filtered water
- Juice of half a lemon (freshly squeezed)
- ¼ to ½ teaspoon of pink Himalayan salt (start with ¼ tsp if you're new to it)
- Optional: a slice of fresh ginger or a dash of raw apple cider vinegar for added digestive support

Stir gently. Sip slowly. Drink it on an empty stomach, ideally within 30 minutes of waking. Wait 15–20 minutes before eating or drinking anything else.

This single ritual triggers:

- Cellular hydration (the salt acts as a transporter, moving water *into* your cells)

- Digestive awakening (lemon and salt stimulate stomach acid and bile flow)

- Adrenal signaling (the salt calms early cortisol spikes that cause belly fat retention)

- Electrolyte balance (especially after night sweating or mineral depletion from stress)

Within 3–5 days, many women report:

- Lighter, flatter stomach upon waking

- Easier bowel movements and less gas

- More stable energy until lunch

- Fewer cravings before noon

- A natural reduction in brain fog

This is not just hydration. It's a reset—from the inside out.

Best Times to Use Salt for Hormonal

45

Signaling

Let's go deeper.

Your body operates on a circadian hormonal clock, and salt plays a role in how effectively those hormones fire. When used at the right times, salt can support better metabolism, mood regulation, and hormone clearance.

Here's how the salt trick pairs with your body's natural hormonal windows:

Morning (6:00 AM – 9:00 AM):

- Cortisol naturally rises to help you wake up.
- This is when salt + lemon water supports adrenal balance, preventing overactivation of stress hormones.
- It also helps trigger thyroid hormone conversion for metabolism.

Midday (12:00 PM – 2:00 PM):

- Blood sugar dips are common. This is when most cravings and energy crashes happen.

- A cup of salted herbal tea can help stabilize glucose and reduce emotional eating.

- The salt here grounds your nervous system, helping prevent spikes in insulin or cortisol.

Evening (8:00 PM – 9:00 PM):

- Melatonin begins to rise, and your body enters repair mode.

- A warm drink with salt + magnesium can soothe the nervous system, improve sleep, and reduce overnight water retention.

- This supports overnight fat-burning, since the liver detox pathways rely on mineral support.

Timing matters. Not just what you eat—but *when and why*.

Hydration for Fat-Burning vs. Water Retention

Hydration is a misunderstood piece of the weight loss puzzle.

Many women drink excessive amounts of plain water, thinking it will "flush fat" or help them lose weight. But here's the truth: plain water without minerals can make you more bloated, not less.

Your cells are electrical. They need minerals—especially sodium, magnesium, potassium, and chloride—to transport water across cell membranes. Without these, water moves through your system without truly hydrating you. You pee it out, lose more minerals, and create a feedback loop of dehydration and water retention.

So what's the solution?

Mineralized hydration.

When you add a pinch of pink salt to your water:

- Your cells absorb the water more efficiently

- Your lymph system drains better (reducing puffiness)

- Your digestion improves (because stomach acid relies on sodium chloride)

- Your metabolism gets a subtle ignition (especially when paired with lemon or cinnamon)

Signs your current hydration isn't working:

- You're always thirsty, yet bloated

- You drink water constantly but still have dry skin or lips

- You wake up puffy despite low sodium intake

- You experience frequent headaches or lightheadedness

Signs your hydration is improving with the salt ritual:

- Your belly feels lighter and flatter

- You urinate less frequently, but more fully

- Your energy is steadier through the day

- Your sugar cravings start to disappear

This is real hydration—and it's critical for releasing weight safely.

The 21-Day Reset Ritual Plan

You don't need a strict food plan or calorie log. You need three anchor points each day that tell your body: *"We are moving toward balance."*

Each ritual serves a different purpose, but together they form a cycle of repair, rhythm, and fat-burning readiness.

Morning Ritual: Pink Salt + Lemon Water

Purpose: Wake up digestion, stimulate metabolism, energize cells, reduce bloating

Best time: Within 30 minutes of waking

Additions: ginger slice (for digestion), cayenne (for thermogenesis), ACV (for insulin sensitivity)

Midday Ritual: Salted Metabolism Tea

Purpose: Prevent energy crashes, stabilize blood sugar, ease afternoon cravings

Best time: After lunch or during your mid-day slump

Tea ideas: peppermint (digestion), cinnamon (insulin), fennel (bloat), turmeric (inflammation)

Additions: 1 pinch pink salt, optional lemon, cinnamon, or dash of honey

Evening Ritual: Salt + Magnesium Calm Drink

Purpose: Calm the nervous system, reduce cortisol, encourage deep sleep and overnight healing

Best time: 30–60 minutes before bed

Recipe: warm water or nut milk + pinch of pink salt + magnesium citrate or glycinate + chamomile, vanilla, or ashwagandha

Each ritual builds on the last. As you repeat this over 21 days, your body begins to relearn trust, safety, and rhythm.

How to Listen to Your Body Daily

Forget apps. Forget calorie calculators.

Your body is giving you real-time feedback every single day. You just need to know how to read it.

Pay attention to:

- **Morning energy**: If you feel groggy or wired, adjust your salt dose or lemon ratio.

- **Midday hunger**: Are you truly hungry or just seeking stimulation? A salt tea may solve it.

- **Cravings**: Do they come in waves? Track them. They often coincide with stress, hormone dips, or poor hydration.

- **Bloat patterns**: If you're more bloated after certain meals, experiment with digestion-boosting rituals.

- **Mood**: Anxiety, irritability, or brain fog are often signs of adrenal strain—mineral replenishment can soothe this.

By checking in, you begin to notice that you're not "crazy" or "lazy." You're underfed in minerals, overstressed, and over-depleted.

This ritual framework brings you back to wholeness.

A Daily Checklist for Alignment

Here's a mental ritual to walk through each day. No pressure—just curiosity:

- Did I start the day with the Pink Salt Morning Elixir?
- Did I pause midday to hydrate with intention?
- Did I eat to nourish—not to escape?
- Did I take five deep breaths at any point today?
- Did I end the day with a calming mineral ritual?

If you miss a day? Grace. If you feel off? Adjust. This isn't about doing it perfectly. It's about building safety, one ritual at a time.

Your Body is a System—Not a Project

This chapter isn't just a guide. It's a turning point.

When you begin to organize your day around support instead of punishment, everything changes. You move from control to care. From fatigue to flow. From weight obsession to metabolic restoration.

And that's where real, sustainable, lifelong weight loss begins.

In the next chapter, we'll explore why this works so well for women—especially those who've struggled with belly fat, hormone shifts, or failed diets. We'll dive into the hormonal blueprint behind fat storage and reveal how this daily ritual helps you burn fat without restriction, stress, or sacrifice.

You're already on the path. Keep sipping.

THE DAILY RITUAL BLUEPRINT
RESET, REHYDRATE, REIGNITE

The Morning Salt Water Ritual

step-by-step with recipe

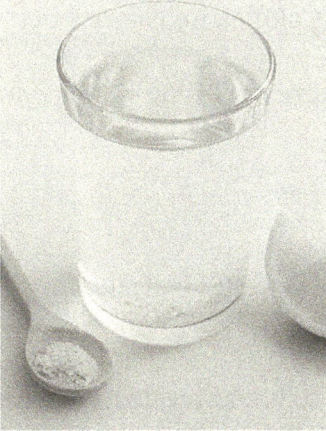

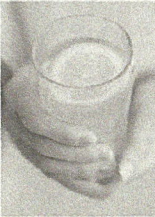

21-Day Reset Ritual Plan

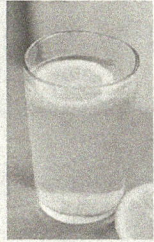

Morning
Salt + lemon water

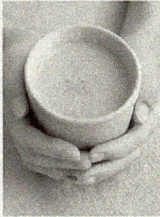

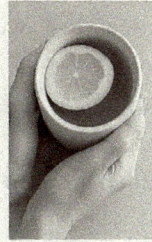

Midday
Salted metabolium tea

Listen to Your Body

- Fatigue
- Cravings
- Bloat

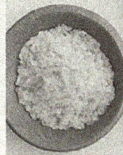

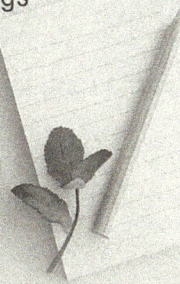

Morning
Salt + lemon water

Evening
Salt + magnesium calm drink

Chapter 3

Fat-Burning Without Dieting — The Hormone Approach

For decades, women have been told that weight loss is a simple formula: eat less, move more. Calories in, calories out. Cut carbs, shrink your portions, and if you're not losing weight, you must not be trying hard enough.

But what if you've been trying—and still feel stuck?

What if you've restricted, tracked, and hustled your way through diet after diet, only to gain the weight back—or worse, feel heavier, more exhausted, and emotionally drained with each attempt?

If this sounds familiar, it's not because you're weak.

It's because your body was never designed to lose weight through deprivation. Your body—especially your hormonal system—has one job above all: to keep you alive, safe, and protected.

And when it senses restriction, stress, or famine, it doesn't burn fat.

It holds on.

That's the hormonal truth most diets ignore. And it's why fat-burning for women must begin with balance—not punishment.

This is where the *Pink Salt Trick* comes in—not as a magical cure, but as a deeply supportive tool that helps restore the very systems dieting has disrupted: your cortisol response, your thyroid hormones, your blood sugar balance, and your adrenal resilience.

Let's unpack this fully—because once you understand how your hormones *actually* work, you'll never fall for toxic diet culture again.

Why Women's Bodies Resist Dieting

To understand why dieting often fails women, we have to first understand what dieting actually is—on a physiological level.

Most diets trigger one or more of the following:

- Calorie restriction

- Carbohydrate elimination

- Fasting windows that override hunger

- Excessive exercise without recovery

- Mental stress around food guilt and control

To the body, these tactics don't register as "health." They register as stress.

And in women—especially women with hormonal fluctuations (PMS, perimenopause, menopause, thyroid imbalances)—that stress has a magnified effect.

Here's what happens:

- **Cortisol rises** in response to perceived threat (even if that threat is just skipping breakfast).

- **Insulin sensitivity drops**, making it harder to process carbohydrates and easier to store fat.

- **Thyroid function slows down**, reducing your resting metabolic rate.

- **Progesterone decreases**, increasing estrogen dominance and belly fat.

- **Cravings increase**, leading to rebound binges or emotional eating.

In short: your body doesn't trust that it's safe to let go of weight. So it clings. Not out of sabotage, but out of survival.

Cortisol, Insulin & Thyroid: The Dieting

Disaster Trio

Let's take a closer look at the three main hormones that get disrupted by restrictive dieting:

1. Cortisol (Your Stress Hormone)

Cortisol is essential for life—it helps you wake up in the morning, respond to emergencies, and regulate inflammation. But when it's chronically elevated (from fasting, overexercising, or emotional stress), it:

- Promotes fat storage, especially in the belly
- Breaks down muscle tissue (lowering your metabolism)
- Disrupts sleep (making cravings worse)
- Increases salt cravings and blood pressure

Cortisol overload is one of the top reasons women hit weight loss plateaus—even when they're "doing everything right."

2. Insulin (Your Blood Sugar Hormone)

Insulin helps shuttle glucose into your cells for energy. But when it's constantly triggered—by stress, erratic eating, or sugar spikes—your cells stop responding efficiently.

This is called insulin resistance, and it leads to:

- Constant hunger and energy crashes

- Fat gain around the midsection

- Difficulty burning fat between meals

- Inflammation and hormone imbalances

Restrictive dieting can worsen insulin resistance, especially if it includes long gaps without nourishment or sugar-filled "cheat days."

3. Thyroid Hormones (Your Metabolism Engine)

Your thyroid controls how fast your body burns calories, maintains energy, and regulates mood and temperature. But it's incredibly sensitive to stress and mineral depletion.

Low-calorie dieting and chronic cortisol:

- Lower *T3*, your active thyroid hormone
- Suppress conversion from T4 to T3
- Lead to fatigue, hair loss, constipation, and weight gain despite clean eating

Which means: you could be eating perfectly... and still gaining weight, simply because your thyroid has downshifted in response to restriction.

Salt's Role in Adrenal Healing & Fat Burning

Now let's talk about salt—the unsung hero of hormonal recovery.

We've been taught to fear salt as the enemy of health. But in reality, *natural pink Himalayan salt* is a foundational tool for hormonal *healing*, especially for women dealing with adrenal fatigue, stress weight, or slow metabolism.

Here's how:

➤ Adrenal Support

Your adrenal glands require *sodium and potassium* to produce aldosterone, which regulates fluid balance and blood pressure. When you're under stress or restricting food, your adrenal function drops—and so does aldosterone. This leads to:

- Salt cravings
- Low blood pressure
- Dizziness or fatigue when standing
- Poor sleep and nighttime waking
- Water retention and bloating

Adding mineral-rich pink salt to your morning ritual replenishes adrenal reserves, helping you regulate hydration, calm cortisol, and reduce salt cravings throughout the day.

➤ Thyroid Boost

Your thyroid uses iodine and sodium to produce T3 and T4 hormones. Without enough of these minerals, conversion slows— and your metabolism stalls. Pink salt provides trace elements that support thyroid function, especially in women with sluggish metabolism.

➤ Fat-Burning Kickstart

Salt also supports bile production, which helps you digest fats and absorb fat-soluble vitamins like A, D, E, and K. Without enough bile, fat metabolism becomes sluggish—and fat loss stalls. A morning salt ritual stimulates bile flow, helping your liver detox more efficiently and your digestive system process healthy fats properly.

In short: pink salt doesn't "cause weight gain." It provides the nutritional safety net your body needs to *let go of stored fat*.

How the Salt Trick Stabilizes Blood Sugar and Hunger

Blood sugar swings are one of the biggest hidden causes of weight gain and chronic fatigue.

Here's the pattern many women experience:

1. Skip breakfast → blood sugar crashes mid-morning

2. Cravings hit → reach for sugar or caffeine

3. Temporary energy boost → insulin spikes

4. Crash again → more cravings

5. Late-night snacking → poor sleep → repeat

The *Pink Salt Trick interrupts this cycle* in a gentle but powerful way.

Here's what it does:

- The *salt + lemon water* first thing in the morning stabilizes cortisol and prevents early blood sugar dips.

- Salt supports insulin sensitivity by helping the pancreas regulate glucose metabolism.

- Pink salt provides minerals like magnesium and chromium, which reduce sugar cravings and stabilize mood.

- Salted teas and snacks throughout the day prevent hypoglycemia crashes, which are often mistaken for hunger.

As a result, your hunger becomes real, not reactive. Your energy stabilizes. Your brain feels clearer. And fat-burning becomes accessible—because your body isn't chasing sugar or reacting to chaos. It's operating in flow.

A Sample Day: No-Diet, Salt-Enhanced Fat-

Burning Schedule

Here's what a day could look like using the Pink Salt Blueprint to promote fat-burning without restriction:

Morning

- Wake up and sip your Pink Salt Morning Elixir (warm water + lemon + ¼ tsp pink salt)
- Wait 20 minutes
- Eat a protein-rich breakfast (e.g., eggs + greens + avocado + sprinkle of salt)
- Light movement: stretching, walking, sunlight exposure

Midday

- Lunch: grilled protein + steamed veggies + healthy fat + sea salt
- Herbal tea with a pinch of pink salt + cinnamon to support digestion

- Brief rest or walk (supports blood sugar balance)

Evening

- Light dinner with complex carbs (e.g., sweet potato, quinoa)

- Hydration: warm magnesium + pink salt tea

- Tech-free wind-down, deep breathing, early sleep

Notice: There's no restriction. No starvation. Just rhythm. Your body is nourished, supported, and reminded at every step: *You are safe to burn fat.*

Real Case Study: How Sarah Lost 12 lbs Without Dieting or the Gym

Let's meet Sarah.

Sarah is 41. She works a full-time job, has two teenage daughters, and had tried every diet you can name: keto, intermittent fasting, plant-based cleanses, 1200-calorie plans. Each one worked briefly—then backfired.

She came across the Pink Salt Trick not through a diet blog, but through a wellness friend who gave her a jar of Himalayan salt and a simple message:

"Try this in your water every morning. Just start there."

Sarah was skeptical. But desperate.

In the first week, she felt less puffy, had a morning bowel movement for the first time in months, and didn't reach for her usual 10 a.m. pastry.

By the end of Week 2, she noticed:

- 3 lbs down
- Less bloating at night
- Energy throughout the day
- Calmer sleep

- Fewer mood swings around her cycle

She didn't change her meals drastically. She just followed the salt rituals—morning elixir, midday metabolism tea, and evening magnesium blend.

Within *five weeks*, she lost *12 lbs*, stopped binge eating at night, and finally felt in sync with her body—not at war with it.

Let This Be Your Turning Point

You don't need another diet.

You need to restore your body's ability to burn fat—*without panic, punishment, or perfection.*

The Pink Salt Trick is not a shortcut. It's a repatterning ritual. It gives your hormones the safety, rhythm, and nourishment they've been missing.

In the next chapter, we'll take this even further—by helping you beat the bloat and repair your digestion using the salt-gut connection. Because fat-burning begins in the gut—and pink salt is the catalyst your digestive system has been waiting for.

Keep going. You're not just losing weight.

You're rebuilding trust.

Fat-Burning Without Dieting — The Hormone Approach

Dieting often fails women due to its effects on hormones. By balancing cortisol, insulin, and tyiroid function, the Pink Salt Trick can help you lose weight naturally.

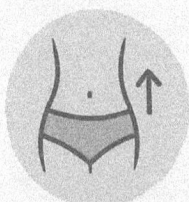

Cortisol Disruption

Chronic stress raises belly fat-storing corisol

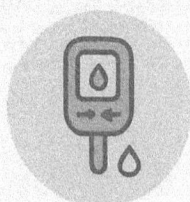

Insulin Resistance

Dieting causes cravings & blood sugar spikes

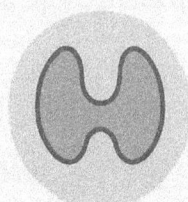

Thyroid Slowdown

Low-calorie diets suppress fat-burning thyroid

How Salt Supports Fat Loss

- Nourishes & calms adrenals
- Improves insulin sensitivity
- Stimulates bile for fat metablism

Sample No-Diet Day

Salt + lemon water, protein breakfast

Sample No-Diet Day

Morning Salt + lemon water, protein breakfast

Midday Salted herbal tea after lunch

Nighttime Sait + magnesium drink

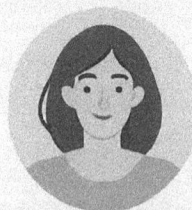

Case Study: Sarah Lost 12 lbs

- Used the Pink Salt Trick daily

72

Chapter 4

Beat the Bloat — Gut Health, Digestion & Debloating Recipes

There's a specific kind of heaviness that doesn't show up on a scale. It's the fullness that creeps in after you've eaten something small and clean—but your stomach still feels swollen, tight, or uncomfortable. It's the kind of discomfort that makes you unbutton your jeans in secret or wake up already feeling "off," before the day even starts.

That's bloating. And for millions of women, it's become so common it feels normal.

But it's not.

Bloating is a signal. It's your body's way of telling you that something in your digestion, hydration, mineral balance, or stress response is out of sync.

The good news? You can reverse it. And one of the fastest, gentlest, and most effective ways to do that isn't a supplement, pill, or restrictive cleanse.

It's salt. More specifically, *pink Himalayan salt*—combined with the right rituals, herbs, and spices to help you debloat naturally and feel light again.

This chapter is your roadmap to understanding why you bloat, how to fix it, and how to make your kitchen a daily gut-healing apothecary. Let's break it all down.

Salt's Role in Bile Production and Gut Acid

Balance

Let's start with the basics: Digestion begins long before food reaches your stomach.

The moment you smell, taste, or think about food, your body prepares to break it down. But in order to digest food properly—especially fats and proteins—you need three critical elements:

1. Sufficient stomach acid

2. Adequate bile production

3. Smooth, rhythmic muscle contractions in the gut

Pink salt supports *all three*.

➤ Stomach Acid Activation

Contrary to popular belief, many cases of bloating, heartburn, and indigestion are caused by too little stomach acid, not too much.

When stomach acid is low, food ferments in the gut, gases form, and the digestion process slows dramatically.

Sodium chloride (the base mineral in salt) is essential for producing hydrochloric acid (HCl), the main acid your stomach uses to break down food. When you don't get enough real salt in your diet—especially if you've been avoiding it—you may experience:

- Constant bloating after meals
- Gas, burping, or fullness after small portions
- Acid reflux (from food backing up due to slow digestion)
- Feeling "stuck" or heavy in your gut

A pinch of pink salt in warm water before meals can gently stimulate HCl production, giving your body the acid it needs to digest food fully and comfortably.

➤ Bile Flow and Fat Digestion

Bile is a golden-green fluid produced by your liver and stored in the gallbladder. Its job is to *emulsify fat,* escort toxins out of the body, and help absorb fat-soluble vitamins like A, D, E, and K.

When bile flow is sluggish, fat digestion slows down. You feel heavy. Your belly inflates. You may get headaches, nausea, or skin breakouts. Many women—even those eating healthy—have sluggish bile due to stress, hormone imbalances, low-fat diets, or mineral deficiencies.

Pink salt helps in two key ways:

- It contains minerals like sodium and chloride needed for optimal bile formation.
- It supports stomach acid, which triggers the gallbladder to release bile on time.

The result? Better fat digestion, smoother elimination, and less bloating after meals—especially when you pair it with digestion-friendly herbs.

Common Bloat Triggers—and How Pink Salt Counteracts Them

Understanding what causes bloating is half the battle. Once you know the triggers, you can create rituals to preempt and neutralize them.

1. Low Stomach Acid

Trigger: Undigested food lingers too long in the gut.

Salt Solution: Sip salt + lemon water 20 minutes before meals.

2. Poor Bile Flow

Trigger: Difficulty digesting fats, fullness after healthy meals.

Salt Solution: Add pink salt to warm lemon-ginger tea to stimulate bile.

3. Dehydration

Trigger: Constipation, dry stool, swollen belly.

Salt Solution: Hydrate with mineral-rich water + pink salt throughout the day.

4. Processed Salt + Sodium Overload

Trigger: Swelling, puffiness from table salt in packaged foods.

Salt Solution: Replace with *pure pink Himalayan salt* only. It nourishes instead of stressing the body.

5. Stress + Shallow Breathing

Trigger: Slowed peristalsis, "nervous belly," bloating before events.

Salt Solution: Combine salt water with *adaptogenic teas* (like holy basil or ashwagandha) to relax gut-brain connection.

6. Fermentation from Sugar + Inflammatory Foods

Trigger: Gas, discomfort, bloating after eating even healthy carbs.

Salt Solution: Use salted herbal teas like fennel or mint to reduce inflammation and balance gut microbes.

In all cases, pink salt acts as a *gut reset.* It restores lost minerals, regulates stomach acid, and partners beautifully with specific herbs to help your body do what it already wants to do: digest well.

The Best Herbs, Teas, and Spices to Pair with

Pink Salt

To turn your salt rituals into powerful *gut-healing elixirs,* pair them with ingredients that soothe, stimulate, or support digestion:

Fennel

Calms intestinal spasms, reduces gas, relieves bloating.

Best paired with: Salted hot tea or digestive shot

Lemon

Stimulates bile and stomach acid, supports liver function.

Best paired with: Morning salt elixir or warm pre-meal tonic

Mint

Relaxes the digestive tract, reduces nausea and bloating.

Best paired with: Midday salted tea or cold flush

Ginger

Speeds up gastric emptying, warms the belly, reduces inflammation.

Best paired with: Lemon–Ginger–Salt Elixir

Chamomile

Soothes gut lining, calms nerves, eases IBS-type discomfort.

Best paired with: Nighttime salt + calm drink

Turmeric

Reduces inflammation and supports liver detox pathways.

Best paired with: Anti-Bloat Broth or morning warm tea

These herbs *amplify the effects of pink salt*, making your debloating rituals faster and more effective—without any side effects.

Debloating Recipes

These are your go-to formulas when your belly feels off, inflamed, or overfull. Each one can be used daily, or rotated as needed. They're fast, effective, and made with ingredients you likely already have.

Lemon–Ginger–Salt Elixir

Purpose: Pre-meal acid booster + morning detox

How to Make:

- 1 cup warm water
- Juice of ½ lemon
- ¼ tsp grated fresh ginger
- ⅛ tsp pink Himalayan salt
- Optional: dash of cayenne

When to Use:

- First thing in the morning

- 15 minutes before a heavy meal

- After a sluggish or bloated day

Why It Works:

Lemon and ginger stimulate stomach acid and bile; salt delivers minerals to support gut flow.

Morning Flat Belly Water

Purpose: All-day hydration with a digestive reset

How to Make:

- 1 liter of filtered water

- ½ cucumber, sliced

- 1 tbsp fresh lemon juice

- 5 fresh mint leaves

- ⅛ tsp pink salt

When to Use:

- Sip throughout the day

- Start with 1 glass after waking

Why It Works:

Combines gentle detox with electrolyte balance and digestive calm.

Mint and cucumber reduce swelling.

Cucumber–Mint–Salt Flush

Purpose: Light, refreshing bloat relief

How to Make:

- 1 glass cold water

- 2 thin cucumber slices

- 3 mint leaves

- Juice of ¼ lime

- Pinch of pink salt

When to Use:

- Hot days, after salty meals, post-bloating episodes

85

Why It Works:

Hydrates and flushes without overloading your kidneys. Helps your lymph system drain excess fluid.

Salted Fennel Digestive Shot

Purpose: Fast gas relief after meals

How to Make:

- ½ cup warm water
- ½ tsp crushed fennel seeds
- ⅛ tsp pink salt
- Optional: drop of raw honey

When to Use:

- Immediately after meals
- Before sleep if digestion feels slow

Why It Works:

Fennel breaks down trapped gas and soothes intestinal inflammation. Salt supports enzyme activation.

Anti-Bloat Broth

Purpose: Deep belly healing and warmth

How to Make:

- 1.5 cups water or vegetable broth
- ½ tsp turmeric
- ¼ tsp grated ginger
- ⅛ tsp pink salt
- Sprinkle of black pepper
- Optional: splash of coconut milk

When to Use:

- Before bed
- On cold days
- When digestion feels stagnant

Why It Works:

This anti-inflammatory blend settles the gut, supports liver detox, and delivers warmth to break down lingering waste.

Bloat-Free Is Your New Normal

Bloating is not something you have to live with. It's not your age, your hormones, or your body type—it's a *correctable imbalance,* and pink salt gives you the power to correct it gently, naturally, and sustainably.

With the right hydration, mineral support, and digestion-loving ingredients, you'll feel the difference not just in your waistline, but in your energy, skin, sleep, and overall ease.

In the next chapter, we'll go deeper into hormone healing—showing you how the Pink Salt Trick supports adrenal, thyroid, and reproductive balance with recipes tailored specifically for *hormonal weight gain, PMS, and mood swings.*

Your belly is softening. Your gut is listening. And your bloat? It's on its way out.

Beat the Bloat
Gut Health, Digestion & Debloating Recipes

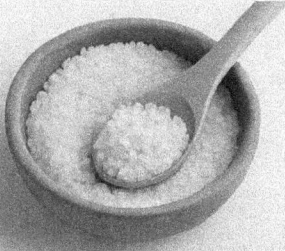

Salt's role in bile production and gut acid balance

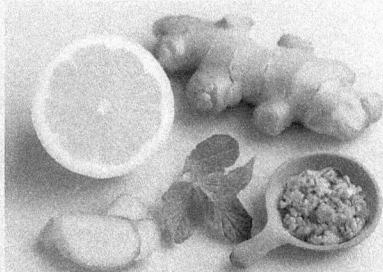

Common bloat triggers and how pink salt counteracts them

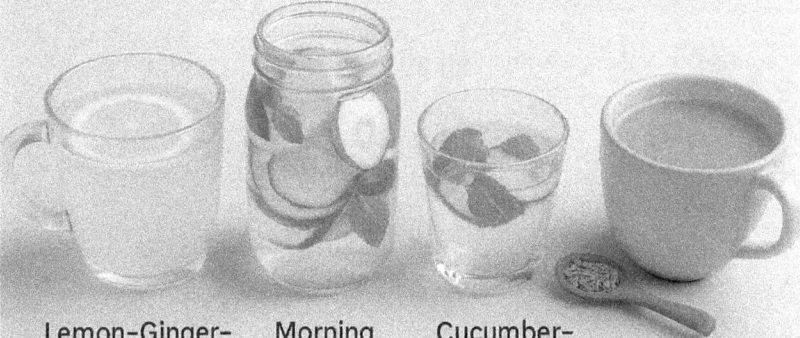

Lemon-Ginger-Salt Elixir

Morning Flat Belly Water

Cucumber-Mint-Salt Flush

Salted Fennl Digestive Shot

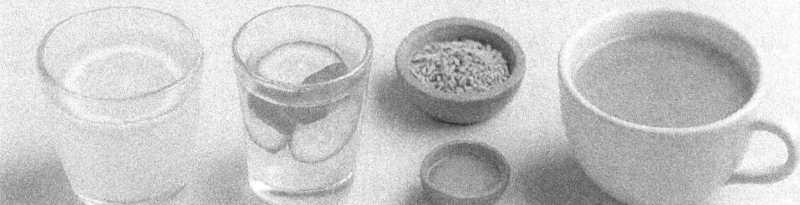

Chapter 5

Hormone Reset Recipes — Adrenal, Thyroid & Mood Support

If weight loss feels harder than it used to... if you're constantly tired, puffy, moody, or wired at night and flatlined in the morning... if your cravings swing wildly and your PMS feels like it's running the show, this chapter is for you.

Because this isn't about willpower.

It's about hormones.

And if your hormones are out of balance—no amount of dieting, exercise, or self-discipline will fix the real issue.

Your body doesn't want to hold onto weight. It's not sabotaging you. It's protecting you—from perceived stress, mineral loss, and internal chaos. That protection shows up as belly fat, sluggish thyroid, mood swings, water retention, and extreme fatigue. But underneath it all is a cry for regulation. For rhythm. For nourishment.

And one of the most overlooked tools in helping you reset your hormones naturally is something humble, mineral-rich, and completely within your reach: *pink Himalayan salt.*

In this chapter, we're going to walk you through:

- Why hormonal weight gain happens, even with healthy habits
- How pink salt nourishes the adrenal-thyroid-reproductive system
- Specific recipes and rituals to reset mood, metabolism, and menstrual balance

Let's start by demystifying the most common hormonal patterns affecting women's weight and energy today.

Hormonal Weight Gain Explained

Women's bodies are beautifully complex—and exquisitely sensitive to change. Your hormones shift daily, weekly, monthly, and across every decade of your life. But in today's world of chronic stress, poor sleep, inflammation, and dietary confusion, many women live in a perpetual state of imbalance.

Let's simplify the most common patterns of hormone-related weight gain:

1. Estrogen Dominance

- Occurs when estrogen levels are too high relative to progesterone
- Causes: hormonal birth control, xenoestrogens (plastics, beauty products), poor liver detox, stress
- Symptoms: PMS, bloating, breast tenderness, fat gain in hips and thighs, irritability

2. Cortisol Spikes

- Occurs when your body is in chronic fight-or-flight

- Causes: overexercising, undereating, poor sleep, emotional stress

- Symptoms: belly fat, anxiety, fatigue, sugar cravings, insomnia

3. Thyroid Slumps

- Occurs when your thyroid slows down its hormone production

- Causes: mineral deficiencies (iodine, selenium, sodium), chronic stress, inflammation

- Symptoms: slow metabolism, cold hands and feet, hair loss, brain fog, constipation

These three patterns often overlap—and they're not "solved" by cutting calories. They're resolved by replenishing, rebalancing, and resetting your endocrine system. And that's where pink salt becomes more than seasoning—it becomes a daily therapeutic ally.

Pink Salt as a Foundational Electrolyte for Hormonal Harmony

Your hormones don't operate in isolation. They are deeply affected by the state of your mineral balance, especially your electrolytes: sodium, potassium, calcium, and magnesium.

Mineral deficiencies—particularly in sodium and magnesium—send stress signals to your adrenal glands. This triggers cortisol production, depletes progesterone, suppresses thyroid function, and destabilizes insulin. The result? Fat storage, fatigue, inflammation, and hormonal chaos.

Pink Himalayan salt helps reverse this spiral by:

- Replenishing sodium and trace minerals required for adrenal function

- Supporting hydration at the cellular level, easing water retention and fatigue

- Providing chloride, which aids in stomach acid production and digestion

- Supporting iodine utilization in the thyroid gland

- Helping the body retain magnesium, which is critical for mood and hormonal regulation

In short: pink salt isn't just for flavor—it's a functional foundation. And when you pair it with the right adaptogens, herbs, and cycle-supporting foods, it becomes a powerful tool for daily hormone healing.

Let's get into the recipes.

Hormone Healing Recipes

Each of these recipes is designed to target a specific aspect of your hormonal landscape—whether you're dealing with cortisol surges, thyroid sluggishness, PMS, cramping, or mood swings.

They're easy to prepare, deeply nourishing, and build on the rituals you've already started with the Pink Salt Trick.

Salted Ashwagandha Honey

Purpose: Adrenal support, anxiety relief, deep sleep

Ingredients:

- 1 tablespoon raw honey
- ½ teaspoon ashwagandha powder
- 1 pinch pink Himalayan salt
- Optional: sprinkle of cinnamon or cardamom

Instructions:

- Mix all ingredients into a paste

- Take 1 teaspoon in the evening before bed

- Allow to dissolve in the mouth or stir into warm herbal tea

Why It Works:

Ashwagandha is an adaptogen that lowers cortisol and nourishes adrenal glands. Combined with pink salt and raw honey, it supports mineral replenishment and relaxes the nervous system, helping restore hormonal balance while you sleep.

Thyroid-Boosting Salt Tonics

Purpose: Reignite metabolism, improve energy, support fat-burning

Tonic #1: Morning Metabolism Spark

- 10 oz warm water

- Juice of ½ lemon

- ¼ teaspoon pink salt

- 1 teaspoon coconut oil or MCT oil

- Optional: a dash of cayenne pepper

Tonic #2: Midday Thyroid Nourish

- 1 cup herbal tea (nettle, dandelion, or green tea)
- ⅛ teaspoon pink salt
- ½ teaspoon kelp or seaweed powder (iodine source)
- Splash of lemon or apple cider vinegar

Why It Works:

These tonics provide the minerals (sodium, iodine, potassium) your thyroid needs to produce hormones efficiently. The healthy fat (MCT oil) supports energy, while the salt improves bile flow, aiding nutrient absorption critical for thyroid health.

PMS-Soothing Pink Salt Latte

Purpose: Balance mood, reduce bloating, ease tension before menstruation

Ingredients:

- 1 cup warm unsweetened almond or oat milk

- 1 teaspoon raw cacao or carob powder

- ¼ teaspoon pink Himalayan salt

- ½ teaspoon maca powder (optional)

- Dash of cinnamon or vanilla

- Natural sweetener (stevia, honey, or date syrup)

Instructions:

- Warm milk in a saucepan

- Whisk in cacao, salt, and powders until smooth

- Sweeten to taste and sip slowly in the evening

Why It Works:

Cacao contains magnesium and mood-elevating compounds. Maca supports hormonal harmony. Salt helps retain these minerals and reduce bloating, especially in the luteal phase of your cycle when estrogen dips and progesterone fluctuates.

Menstrual Cramp Relief Water

Purpose: Soothe cramps, reduce water retention, promote uterine relaxation

Ingredients:

- 12 oz warm filtered water
- Juice of ½ lemon
- ⅛ teaspoon pink Himalayan salt
- ¼ teaspoon powdered ginger or turmeric
- Optional: a pinch of black pepper

Instructions:

- Mix and sip slowly, especially during cramping
- Can be repeated every 4–6 hours as needed

Why It Works:

Ginger and turmeric reduce inflammation. Pink salt helps regulate water balance and muscle contractions. The result? A natural alternative to NSAIDs or over-the-counter painkillers, with added hormonal benefit.

Salted Seed-Cycling Blends

Purpose: Balance estrogen and progesterone throughout your menstrual cycle

Seed-Cycling Basics:

- Days 1–14 (Follicular Phase): 1 tbsp ground flax + 1 tbsp ground pumpkin seeds

- Days 15–28 (Luteal Phase): 1 tbsp ground sunflower + 1 tbsp sesame seeds

- Add 1 small pinch of pink salt to each daily serving

How to Use:

- Stir into smoothies, yogurt, oatmeal, or nut milk

- Keep refrigerated to preserve nutrients

- Take daily in the corresponding phase of your cycle

Why It Works:

Seeds contain lignans and essential fatty acids that help modulate estrogen and support progesterone production. Salt enhances absorption and supports the liver in processing hormones, making seed-cycling more effective.

You Can Reset—Gently, Naturally, Daily

You don't need a hormonal crash course or prescription protocol to feel like yourself again.

You need consistency, minerals, and gentle nourishment that matches the rhythms of your body.

Pink salt is more than a tool for digestion or hydration. It is a hormone ally—quietly and powerfully supporting your thyroid, adrenals, reproductive cycle, and mood through every phase of your month and life.

As you begin incorporating these recipes, listen to your body. Notice what shifts. Track your sleep, cravings, energy, and mood—not out of control, but out of curiosity and care.

In the next chapter, we'll explore how to use pink salt to fight inflammation from the inside out, reduce cravings, and stabilize energy by integrating anti-inflammatory eating principles.

This journey isn't about fixing your body. It's about finally working with it.

Hormone Reset Recipes

– Adrenal, Thyroid & Mood Support

Hormonal weight gain, fatigue, cravings and mood swings aren't signs of lack of willpower. They are messages that your hormones need support, not restriction—and simple ingredients like pink salt can help you reset.

Hormonal Weight Gain Explained

- Estrogen dorninance
  High estrogen & locss; bloating

- Thyroid slumps
  Sluggish metabolism

- Cortisol spikes
  Belly fat & cravings

Pink Salt as a Foundational Electrolyte for Hormonal Harmony

- Stress & adrenal balance
  Helps stress & adrenals

- Hydration & magnesium absorption

- Iodine & thyroid function

Recipes for Hormonal Healing

- Salted Ashwagandha Honey
  1 1 bsp raw honev, fs tsp aswagandha
  pinch of pink salt

- Thyroid-Boosting Salt Tonics
  Tonic 1: warm lemon water • pink sat. :)
  Tonic 2: herbal tea • kelp powder ✗

- PMS-Soothing Pink Salt Latte
  1 cup warm milk: 1 tsp caceo powder
)s tsp pink salt:)1 tsp maca powder
  Combine & whisk:

- Salted Seed-Cycling Blends
  Days 1-14-1 tbsp ground tlax ₹
  1 tbsp ground pumpkin seeds
  • pink salf:
  Days 15-28-1 tbsp ground
  sunflower seeds • 1 tbsp gound sesame

Chapter 6

Anti-Inflammatory Eating with Pink Salt — No More Cravings or Crashes

If you've ever felt like your body is inflamed, heavy, puffy, or constantly "on edge"—even when you're eating clean—there's a good chance chronic inflammation is at the root.

And when inflammation lingers below the surface, it doesn't just affect how you feel. It shapes how your body stores fat, how your hormones behave, how your metabolism runs, how your brain thinks, and whether or not you have the energy to show up in your life.

Inflammation is the silent cause of weight gain, fatigue, cravings, mood swings, and immune dysfunction. But the good news is: you don't need an extreme elimination diet or a detox kit to start calming it.

Sometimes, healing begins with a single mineral—and a shift in how you season your food.

In this chapter, we'll explore:

- Why inflammation blocks weight loss and drains your energy
- How *pink Himalayan salt* reduces gut-based inflammation naturally
- How to cook with pink salt to turn every meal into medicine
- Simple anti-inflammatory recipes you can start using immediately to restore balance, end cravings, and energize your body

Let's begin where most inflammation begins: your gut.

Inflammation: The Hidden Root of Weight

Gain & Fatigue

Inflammation is your body's natural defense mechanism. When you cut yourself, catch a virus, or eat something harmful, your immune system releases chemicals to protect you. This is acute inflammation—and it's helpful.

But when your body stays in a chronic, low-grade inflammatory state—triggered by stress, processed foods, blood sugar spikes, poor sleep, environmental toxins, and digestive imbalances—it becomes destructive.

Here's what chronic inflammation does behind the scenes:

- Raises cortisol and insulin, causing fat to accumulate around your belly
- Slows your thyroid, dragging down your metabolism
- Disrupts leptin and ghrelin, making it harder to feel full or stop eating

- Creates brain fog, mood instability, and a constant craving for sugar

- Damages the gut lining, leading to food sensitivities, bloating, and fatigue

Even women who eat mostly clean and exercise regularly can carry hidden inflammation—especially when stress is high or gut health has been overlooked.

This is where food becomes your medicine—and pink salt becomes a daily tool for reducing the inflammation that's holding your body back.

The Salt–Gut–Inflammation Connection

Most people have been taught to fear salt. But it's not salt that causes inflammation—it's the wrong kind of salt paired with an inflamed gut environment.

Table salt—heavily processed, stripped of minerals, and loaded with anti-caking agents—exacerbates inflammation and contributes to water retention and metabolic stress.

But unrefined pink Himalayan salt does the opposite.

Here's how it supports a calmer, cleaner, and more anti-inflammatory internal environment:

1. It restores electrolyte balance.

Inflammation increases the demand for minerals like magnesium, sodium, and potassium. Pink salt provides over 80 trace minerals that help rebalance the body's electrical and cellular function—especially in the digestive and immune systems.

2. It supports gut lining repair.

Minerals in pink salt, including zinc and selenium, are essential for rebuilding the intestinal wall—reducing the permeability ("leaky gut") that contributes to systemic inflammation.

3. It aids stomach acid and bile production.

Better digestion means less fermentation, less bloating, and fewer immune responses to food—key in reducing gut-triggered inflammation.

4. It supports detoxification and lymphatic flow.

Salt helps the body maintain proper hydration, which is essential for flushing toxins and reducing the burden on the liver and lymph system—two primary hubs for inflammation control.

When used daily—in the right way—pink salt becomes a silent healer, calming internal fires and setting the stage for steady energy, clarity, and natural weight loss.

Now let's bring that healing to your kitchen.

How to Cook with Pink Salt for Anti-

Inflammatory Benefits

Cooking with pink salt doesn't just mean sprinkling it over your meal at the end. It's about infusing your food with mineral support, using it as a *functional ingredient* that elevates flavor and wellness at the same time.

Here are a few smart ways to use pink salt in an anti-inflammatory kitchen:

- Add a pinch to your morning lemon water or herbal tea to support mineral absorption
- Use it to season healthy fats like avocado, olive oil, and nuts (salt helps your body metabolize fats better)
- Combine it with anti-inflammatory spices like turmeric, cinnamon, and cumin in soups or stews
- Mix into smoothies, chia puddings, or seed blends to improve electrolyte balance and flavor

- Sprinkle over roasted vegetables after baking to retain the mineral complexity and crisp texture

- Add to homemade bone broths, herbal drinks, or fermented foods to enhance gut repair

When paired with anti-inflammatory foods—leafy greens, omega-3s, herbs, clean proteins—pink salt becomes a healing catalyst, not just a seasoning.

Quick Anti-Inflammatory Meals & Snacks with Pink Salt

Below are five powerful, flavorful, and craving-busting recipes designed to reduce inflammation, increase energy, and satisfy your body without sugar crashes or bloating.

Salted Avocado Super Toast

Why It Works: Healthy fats + minerals = blood sugar balance + long-lasting energy

How to Make:

- 1 slice sprouted or gluten-free toast
- ½ ripe avocado, mashed
- 1 small pinch pink salt
- Squeeze of lemon
- Sprinkle of turmeric, black pepper, or hemp seeds

When to Eat: Breakfast, mid-morning snack, or light lunch

Benefits: Curbs cravings, stabilizes blood sugar, and provides healthy fat for hormone regulation and brain clarity.

Warm Turmeric–Salt Broth

Why It Works: Anti-inflammatory gold in a cup—soothes joints, gut, and mood

113

How to Make:

- 1.5 cups hot water or bone broth

- ¼ teaspoon turmeric

- 1 pinch pink salt

- Dash of black pepper (to activate curcumin in turmeric)

- Optional: splash of coconut milk or ghee

When to Drink: Mid-afternoon or evening to beat inflammation bloat and calm the body

Benefits: Turmeric reduces joint and cellular inflammation. Pink salt replenishes minerals and supports detoxification.

Salted Green Smoothie Bowl

Why It Works: Combines alkalizing greens, fiber, and minerals for anti-inflammatory detox

How to Make:

- ½ frozen banana

- Handful of spinach or kale

- ½ avocado

- 1 tablespoon chia seeds

- 1 scoop plant-based protein

- Splash of almond milk

- Pinch of pink salt

- Optional: cinnamon, ginger, or mint for flavor

Blend until thick. Pour into a bowl and top with:

- Sliced cucumber

- Hemp seeds

- Fresh mint

- Light drizzle of lemon or olive oil

When to Eat: Post-workout, light breakfast, or inflammation reset meal

Benefits: Combats oxidative stress, supports digestion, and keeps blood sugar steady without sugar spikes.

Seaweed & Salt Mineral Salad

Why It Works: Rich in iodine, magnesium, and electrolytes—supports thyroid and detox

How to Make:

- 1 cup mixed greens

- 1 sheet nori or wakame seaweed, torn

- 1 tablespoon pumpkin seeds

- 1 teaspoon sesame oil or olive oil

- Squeeze of lemon

- Small pinch of pink salt

- Optional: grated carrot, cucumber, or avocado slices

When to Eat: Lunch or dinner side

Benefits: Provides minerals critical for anti-inflammatory hormone function. Salt enhances the absorption of seaweed nutrients.

Salted Chia Pudding for Energy

Why It Works: Fights sugar cravings, balances hormones, fuels muscles and brain

How to Make:

- 2 tablespoons chia seeds
- ¾ cup unsweetened almond milk
- 1 pinch pink salt
- ½ teaspoon vanilla
- Optional: cinnamon, cacao, or maca
- Sweeten with stevia or 1 tsp honey if needed

Let sit overnight or for at least 30 minutes. Top with:

- Sliced berries
- Coconut flakes
- Crushed walnuts or almonds

When to Eat: Mid-morning snack, pre-workout fuel, or late-night craving fix

Benefits: High in omega-3s, fiber, and protein—salt balances blood sugar and helps you absorb nutrients more effectively.

Your Crashes Are Not a Character Flaw — They're a Signal

If you find yourself reaching for sugar, caffeine, or carbs just to get through the day, your body isn't betraying you.

It's *communicating with you*—asking for minerals, hydration, balance, and anti-inflammatory support.

With these meals and rituals, you'll begin to experience:

- Fewer energy dips
- Calmer hunger cues
- Reduced bloating

- Clearer skin

- Improved mood and focus

- Real, sustainable weight release—without obsession

You don't need another restrictive diet. You need nutrient-dense simplicity.

And with pink salt as your healing base, your food becomes a message to your body: *"You are supported. You don't have to hold on anymore."*

In the next chapter, we'll go even deeper by exploring how pink salt can end emotional eating, reduce nervous system stress, and reset your relationship with food through calming rituals and nervous system nourishment.

This isn't just a change in diet. It's a change in how you feel—on every level.

ANTI-INFLAMMATORY EATING WITH PINK SALT

No More Cravings or Crashes

Inflammation: The Root of Weight Gain & Fatigue

- Inflammation raises cortisol, insulin & hunger

The Salt-Gut-Inflammation Connection

- Restores mineral & electrolyte balance
- Aids gut lining repair
- Supports detoxification

How to Cook with Pink Salt

- Season healthy fats & greens
- Combine with anti-inflammatory spices
- Mix into smoothies, chia pudding, etc.

Quick Anti-Inflammatory Meals & Snacks

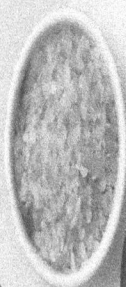

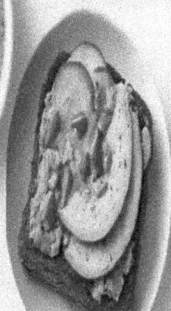

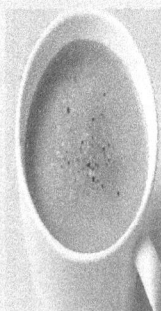

Salted Avocado Super Toast

Warm Turmeric-Salt Broth

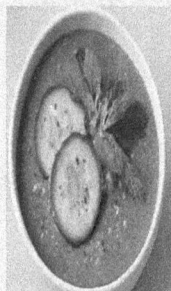

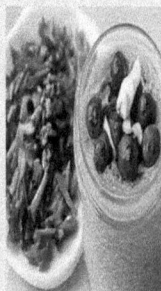

Seaweed & Salt Mineral Salad

Salted Chia Pudding for Energy

Chapter 7

Craving Rescue Recipes — Salt as a Natural Appetite Balancer

It's 3:00 p.m. You had a decent lunch, you're not *really* hungry, but suddenly… you need something sweet. Or salty. Or creamy. Or crunchy. Or maybe it's 10:30 p.m. and you're standing in the kitchen, hunting through the cabinets like a woman possessed, chasing the perfect bite that will finally "do it."

This isn't weakness.

It's biology.

And it's speaking to you—loudly—through cravings.

Cravings aren't just about willpower or emotional eating. More often than not, they're about mineral imbalances, blood sugar instability, and adrenal burnout—and your body trying to fix all three the fastest way it knows how.

This chapter is about understanding where cravings really come from, how pink salt helps reset your natural appetite cues, and how to create delicious, simple recipes that satisfy your brain *and* your body—without triggering more crashes or weight gain.

Let's start with the truth about cravings that no diet will ever tell you.

How Cravings Are Linked to Mineral Imbalances

Your body is incredibly wise. When it craves something, it's often because a deeper nutrient or nervous system need isn't being met.

Craving sugar?

You may be low in magnesium, chromium, or sodium, all of which regulate blood sugar and energy production.

Craving salt?

Your adrenal glands may be depleted, calling for sodium to regulate stress hormones and fluid balance.

Craving chocolate or coffee?

You're likely running on adrenal fatigue, needing magnesium, potassium, or a cortisol spike to feel alive again.

When minerals are low, the body starts reaching for fast fuel:

- **Sugar** to spike dopamine
- **Caffeine** to override fatigue
- **Carbs** to compensate for low serotonin
- **Salty snacks** to try and stabilize low blood pressure

But these fixes are short-lived. They lead to:

- Blood sugar crashes

- Emotional eating spirals

- Mood swings and more cravings

- Fatigue and eventual weight gain

This is where pink salt becomes a craving antidote—because it nourishes the very systems that are being hijacked by these urges.

Using Pink Salt to Stop Sugar, Carb & Caffeine Cravings

Pink Himalayan salt doesn't just make food taste better—it supports the mineral foundation of your body and brain.

Here's how it works against cravings:

1. Replenishes Sodium

Sodium is essential for adrenal health, fluid balance, and electrical communication in the brain. When you're stressed or fatigued, sodium levels drop—and cravings rise. Pink salt restores this balance gently.

2. Enhances Hydration

Dehydration mimics hunger. Pink salt helps your cells absorb water better, easing cravings that are really thirst signals in disguise.

3. Stabilizes Blood Sugar

Salt supports insulin sensitivity and helps maintain more even energy—reducing your need for quick sugar highs.

4. Provides Trace Minerals

Unlike refined salt, pink salt contains over 80 trace minerals that the brain and nervous system depend on to regulate mood, energy, and appetite.

5. Triggers Satisfaction

There's something deeply satisfying about the right balance of sweet and salt. It calms the brain, completes the flavor profile, and creates true satiety.

So instead of fighting your cravings… what if you *fed them*— wisely?

Let's explore five powerful recipes that do just that.

CRAVING-RESET RECIPES

Each recipe below is designed to satisfy a common craving trigger— while nourishing the root cause. They're fast, functional, and absolutely delicious.

Pink Salt Cinnamon Apple Tea

Craving Target: Warm, sweet comfort—midday or after dinner

Why It Works: Apples balance blood sugar. Cinnamon helps regulate insulin. Pink salt supports adrenal function and satisfaction.

How to Make:

- 1 cup hot water
- ½ apple, thinly sliced
- 1 cinnamon stick or ¼ tsp ground cinnamon
- Small pinch of pink salt
- Optional: ½ tsp raw honey

Simmer the apple slices and cinnamon in water for 5 minutes. Add salt and sweetener if needed. Sip slowly while warm.

When to Use:

After meals, during the evening wind-down, or as a dessert substitute.

Sweet-Salt Chocolate Energy Bites

Craving Target: Chocolate, PMS snacks, emotional munchies

Why It Works: Raw cacao contains magnesium and mood-elevating compounds. Pink salt completes the flavor and curbs sugar spikes.

How to Make:

- 1 cup medjool dates, pitted
- ¼ cup raw cacao powder
- ½ cup almonds or walnuts
- 2 tbsp chia seeds or flaxseed
- ¼ tsp pink salt
- 1 tsp vanilla extract
- Optional: coconut flakes or mini dark chocolate chips

Pulse all ingredients in a food processor. Roll into small bites. Store chilled.

When to Use:

Mid-afternoon energy crash, before menstruation, or late-night cravings.

Salted Date Energy Shake

Craving Target: Coffee, sweet drinks, emotional recharging

Why It Works: Dates provide natural sweetness and potassium. Pink salt enhances hydration and deep cellular energy.

How to Make:

- 1 cup unsweetened almond or coconut milk

- 2 medjool dates

- 1 tbsp almond butter

- ¼ tsp pink salt

- ½ tsp cinnamon

- Optional: ice, vanilla, or protein powder

Blend until creamy. Drink slowly to allow minerals to fully absorb.

When to Use:

Morning or midday when reaching for caffeine or sugary lattes.

Salt + Lemon Gummy Snacks

Craving Target: Chewy, tangy, sweet-salty cravings (like candy or sour gummies)

Why It Works: These gummies satisfy texture-based cravings while providing collagen (for gut, skin, and joints) and salt for electrolyte balance.

How to Make:

- ½ cup fresh lemon juice
- 2 tbsp raw honey or maple syrup
- ¼ tsp pink salt
- 2 tbsp grass-fed gelatin powder
- Optional: pinch of turmeric or ginger

Warm the lemon juice and sweetener in a saucepan (don't boil). Stir in gelatin and salt. Pour into silicone molds or a glass container. Chill until set.

When to Use:

Midday slump, PMS snack cravings, or when trying to avoid processed candy.

Coconut-Salt Electrolyte Bark

Craving Target: Sweet-salty chocolate, crunch, salty-fatty snacks

Why It Works: Coconut and cacao deliver healthy fat and antioxidants. Salt brings it into balance for brain and adrenal support.

How to Make:

- ½ cup melted coconut oil
- ¼ cup unsweetened shredded coconut
- 2 tbsp cacao powder
- 1 tbsp maple syrup or monk fruit sweetener
- ¼ tsp pink salt
- Optional: chopped nuts or dried berries

Mix all ingredients. Spread thin on parchment paper. Freeze until solid. Break into shards.

When to Use:

Post-dinner treat, afternoon emotional craving, or healthy snack stash.

Rewiring Cravings is About Nourishing the Need Beneath Them

When your cravings strike, they're not betraying you—they're communicating something:

- "I'm tired and depleted."

- "I need minerals and stable blood sugar."

- "I'm stressed and seeking grounding."

- "I need comfort without consequence."

These recipes answer those calls.

They speak the language of your nervous system—gently rebalancing what's been out of sync through a simple, delicious ritual.

With pink salt as the balancing point, you don't just satisfy your appetite—you reset the pattern of your body and brain.

In the next chapter, we'll build on this even further by exploring how to use 21 days of structured pink salt rituals to create complete transformation—physically, emotionally, and metabolically.

This is your new rhythm.

Cravings don't control you anymore. You've finally found what you were really hungry for all along: mineral-rich nourishment that truly satisfies.

Craving Rescue Recipes

SALT AS A NATURAL APPETITE BALANCER

Craving-Reset Recipes

- How cravings are linked to mineral imbalances
- Using pink salt to stop sugar, carb, and caffeine cravings

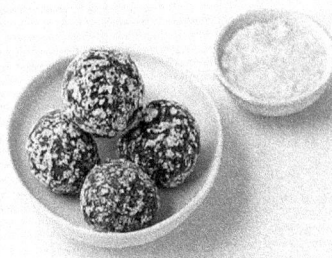

Sweet-Salt Chocolate Energy Bites

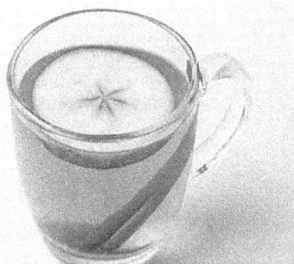

Pink Salt Cinnamon Apple Tea

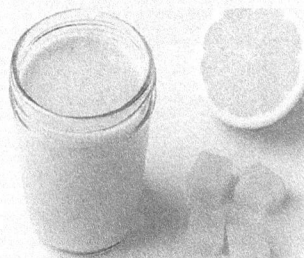

Salt + Lemon Gummy Snacks

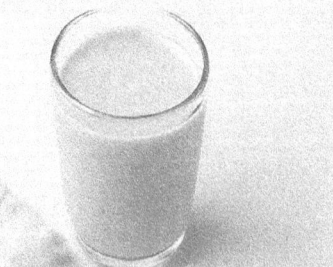

Salted Date Energy Shake

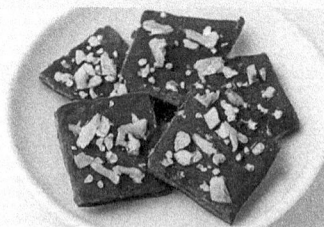

Coconut-Salt Electrolyte Bark

Chapter 8

The 21-Day Pink Salt Reset Plan

Heal Inflammation, Burn Fat, and Balance Hormones Naturally

What if you didn't need to diet, deprive, or obsess to feel like yourself again? What if, instead of "trying harder," you simply aligned your body with a natural rhythm — one that spoke the same biological language as your metabolism, hormones, and nervous system?

That's the purpose of the 21-Day Pink Salt Reset Plan — a rhythm-reset that uses simple mineral rituals, small daily tweaks, and an understanding of your body's real cravings to gently guide you back to balance.

This is not a detox in the extreme sense. You will not starve. You will not restrict. You will reconnect.

Let's begin.

The Rhythm of Reset: Why 21 Days?

Why 21 days? Because habit and healing need rhythm — not pressure. This time frame allows your body to:

- Rehydrate at a cellular level

- Regulate cortisol and blood sugar naturally

- Improve digestion and reduce bloating

- Ease PMS and perimenopause symptoms

- Kickstart sustained fat-burning without dieting

Each week in this plan serves a different metabolic and hormonal purpose.

WEEK 1: Drain the Bloat

"Before fat-burning comes flow."

This is your flush and foundation week. Think of it as unclogging the pipes. Water retention, sluggish digestion, and toxic bloat often mask themselves as "weight." This week gently reverses that.

Goals:

- Reduce excess water retention and puffiness
- Stimulate bile flow and stomach acid naturally
- Restore hydration at the intracellular level

Core Rituals:

- **Wake-Up Salt Tonic**: Pink salt + lemon + warm water = digestive wake-up call.

- **Afternoon Detox Water**: Add cucumber, mint, and a pinch of salt. Sip slowly. Feel lighter.

- **Evening Mineral Calm Mix**: Pink salt + magnesium + warm tea. Relaxes muscles, supports elimination, and improves sleep.

WEEK 2: Fire Up Fat-Burn

"You're not lazy — you're depleted."

Now that your digestion and hydration are aligned, your body is ready to tap into stored energy. This week focuses on reviving the adrenal-thyroid-liver triad — the metabolic powerhouses behind fat-burning.

Goals:

- Support cortisol rhythms (without coffee abuse)
- Activate the thyroid gently
- Reignite energy levels from food, not cravings

Core Rituals:

- **Morning Salt Tonic** (with cayenne or ginger for thermogenesis)

- **Mid-Morning Salt Tea**: Green tea + cinnamon + salt + lemon = blood sugar support + metabolism

- **Salted Protein Add-Ins**: Sprinkle salt on avocado, eggs, or smoothies — it stimulates bile and helps you break down fats better

WEEK 3: Balance the Hormones

"Your hormones are not the enemy — they're messengers."

This is the recalibration phase — the most important for women dealing with hormonal fluctuations, PMS, perimenopause, or weight gain with no clear trigger.

Goals:

- Soothe adrenal fatigue

- Balance estrogen and progesterone naturally

- Calm mood, reduce anxiety, and stabilize hunger cues

Core Rituals:

- **Salt + Seed Cycling Add-Ons** (chia, flax, pumpkin with pink salt)

- **Salted Adaptogenic Tonics** (ashwagandha, holy basil, maca + salt in tea or warm milk)

- **Evening Mineral Calm**: A consistent routine helps your circadian clock and hormone clearance via the liver

DAILY RITUAL TEMPLATE (Use This All 3

Weeks)

Here's your rhythm. You don't have to be perfect — just consistent.

Wake-Up (Within 30 Minutes of Rising)

Salt Tonic:

- 10 oz warm water
- Juice of ½ lemon
- ⅛ tsp pink Himalayan salt
- Optional: pinch of ginger or cayenne

Purpose: Hydrates cells, stimulates digestion, balances cortisol upon waking

Mid-Morning (9:30–11:00 am)

Salt Tea:

- Green or ginger tea

- Slice of apple or cinnamon stick

- ⅛ tsp salt

- Splash of lemon

Purpose: Fights cravings, balances blood sugar, supports thyroid and adrenal flow.

Afternoon (2:00–4:00 pm)

Detox Water:

- 16 oz filtered water

- Cucumber slices, mint leaves, dash of apple cider vinegar

- Small pinch of salt

Purpose: Reduces bloating, supports liver function, beats the slump

Evening (After Dinner or Before Bed)

Mineral Calm Mix:

- Chamomile, rooibos, or magnesium drink

- ⅛ tsp pink salt stirred in

- Optional: drop of lavender or vanilla

Purpose: Soothes nervous system, replenishes minerals lost in the day, promotes restful sleep

PERSONALIZE YOUR RESET

This plan isn't rigid. It breathes with you. Here's how to adapt for unique situations:

PMS or Hormonal Swings:

- Add seed-cycling support with sunflower, pumpkin, or flax

- Increase magnesium-rich foods (dark greens, cacao, nuts — with a salt sprinkle)

- Try the Pink Salt Latte before bed (see Chapter 5) to reduce cramps and tension

Menopause or Perimenopause:

- Swap green tea for holy basil or red clover infusions in the Salt Tea

- Use electrolyte-rich coconut water + salt post hot flashes

- Avoid caffeine in afternoon; rely on pink salt + citrus hydration instead

Energy Slumps or Burnout:

- Sip Salted Apple Cider Vinegar tonic (1 tbsp ACV + 1/8 tsp salt + water)

- Prioritize protein + pink salt in breakfast

- Take 10-minute walks post-meal to help digestion and energy flow

Plateau or Stagnation:

- Revisit Week 1's bloat-release rituals

- Add short bursts of movement (rebounding, breathwork, walking)

- Try alternate-day "power tonics" with extra ginger or cayenne

BONUS: Your 21-Day Reset Tracker & Reflection Journal (Printable)

To help you stay consistent, we've created a daily printable tracker that includes:

- Ritual checkboxes (morning–evening)
- Craving/mood/cramp notes
- Bloat scale and digestion feedback

- 2-minute reflection prompts (What felt good today? What needs love tomorrow?)

Journaling is not about perfection — it's about listening to the body's whispers before they become screams. You'll find the printable PDF in the Bonus Section.

A Closing Word: You're Not Broken — You're Rebalancing

You don't need to fix yourself. You need to refill yourself.

The Pink Salt Reset is not a detox — it's a dialogue with your body. And in 21 days, you'll feel it: your bloat gone, your mood steadier, your cravings reduced, your energy more predictable.

Most of all, you'll feel trust return — not just in pink salt, but in you.

Let's continue this journey together in the next chapter, where we'll explore how to stay light, strong, and balanced long after the reset ends.

21-Day Pink Salt Reset Tracker & Daily Reflection Journal

Your Personal Guide to Listening, Tracking, and Trusting Your Body

DAILY TRACKER TEMPLATE (Print 21 Copies)

Date: _____

Morning Ritual

-

Mid-Morning

-

Afternoon

-

Evening

-

SYMPTOM CHECKLIST (Daily)

•

REFLECTION PROMPT (2 Minutes)

Complete these short prompts each evening.

1. Today I felt most alive when:

_____

2. One thing my body told me today:

_____

3. Tomorrow, I want to feel more:

_____

4. A kind word I want to speak to myself is:

_____

_____

WEEKLY RESET REVIEW (Complete Every 7 Days)

WEEK #: _____

1. How has my energy changed?

_____

2. What physical symptoms have improved (or worsened)?

_____

3. What rituals helped me the most this week?

_____

4. What surprised me about this journey so far?

_____

5. What will I focus on next week?

_____

_____

TIP: Keep your tracker somewhere visible — fridge, bathroom mirror, or bedside table — and take 5 minutes morning and night. This is about connection, not perfection.

You are not on a cleanse. You are on a reclamation.

Chapter 9

Targeted Salt Rituals by Symptom & Goal

You don't need to overhaul your entire life to feel better. Sometimes, you just need to respond to your body's whispers before they become screams.

This chapter is about tuning in, not pushing through. Each of the following rituals is a gentle, natural nudge designed to meet you where you are: tired, bloated, craving sugar, sleepless, or emotionally off-balance. Here, salt becomes your signal partner—a mineral messenger paired with nature's helpers to bring your system back to harmony.

For Belly Bloat: Salt + Digestive Spice Blends

When your stomach feels tight, gassy, or sluggish after meals, your digestion may need a reset. Pink salt, combined with warming spices, can support bile flow, ease gas, and enhance nutrient absorption.

Mini-Ritual:

- 1 cup warm water
- ½ tsp pink salt
- ¼ tsp ground ginger
- A pinch of cumin + fennel seeds (optional)
- Squeeze of lemon juice

Sip slowly before or after meals. This blend encourages digestive fire, reduces fermentation in the gut, and helps the stomach empty more efficiently.

For Low Energy: Pink Salt + Vitamin C Combos

Fatigue that hits midday? It might be more than just sleep. Adrenal stress and low minerals play a huge role. Salt and vitamin C work synergistically to feed your adrenal glands and restore energy.

Mini-Ritual:

- 1 glass spring water
- ½ tsp pink salt
- Juice of ½ orange or lemon
- 1 tsp camu camu powder or acerola cherry (high natural vitamin C)

Use this as a mid-morning or early afternoon recharge tonic. You'll often feel clearer within minutes.

For Sugar Cravings: Electrolyte Fix Tonics

That sudden chocolate craving after lunch? It's often a cry for minerals, not dessert. Electrolytes like sodium, potassium, and magnesium regulate insulin and hunger hormones.

Mini-Ritual:

- 1 cup cold coconut water
- ½ tsp pink salt
- Splash of lime juice
- Optional: sprinkle of cinnamon to curb blood sugar spikes

This salty-sweet balance satisfies your body's deeper needs, not just your tastebuds.

For PMS Or Menopause: Magnesium + Salt

Elixirs

When your hormones swing, your mood, sleep, cravings, and bloating swing too. Magnesium calms the nervous system, while salt anchors hydration and nerve signaling.

Mini-Ritual:

- 1 cup warm almond or oat milk
- ½ tsp pink salt
- 1 tsp magnesium glycinate powder
- Dash of nutmeg or lavender

Sip slowly in the evening, during your luteal phase or any hormonal flare-up. It soothes both physical tension and emotional sensitivity.

For Water Retention: Diuretic Herb + Salt

Pairings

Holding water in your ankles, belly, or fingers? Paradoxically, increasing salt (the right kind) can help—especially when paired with natural diuretics that stimulate kidney flow.

Mini-Ritual:

- 1 cup dandelion tea or parsley tea (steeped 5-7 mins)
- ¼ tsp pink salt
- Slice of cucumber or lemon

Drink in the morning to help flush excess water without depleting electrolytes.

For Mood Swings: Adaptogen + Salt Calming

Brews

Emotional ups and downs are often rooted in blood sugar swings, dehydration, or nervous system dysregulation. Salt stabilizes; adaptogens rewire resilience.

Mini-Ritual:

- 1 cup warm water
- ½ tsp pink salt
- ½ tsp ashwagandha or holy basil (tulsi)
- Dash of cinnamon or clove

Use during emotional lows or high-stress days. It nourishes the vagus nerve and reduces the cortisol cascade.

For Poor Sleep: Evening Salt-Lavender

Infusions

Waking up at 2am? Can't fall asleep despite exhaustion? It may be a mineral drop triggering your cortisol to spike. This infusion helps gently lower cortisol and restore calm.

Mini-Ritual:

- 1 cup warm water or chamomile tea
- ½ tsp pink salt
- ½ tsp dried lavender or lavender tea bag
- Optional: teaspoon of raw honey for blood sugar support

Drink 30 minutes before bed, ideally with no screen time and gentle breathing. Your nervous system will feel hugged.

Note: You don't need a different diet every month. You need a body you can understand and trust. These rituals aren't rules. They're invitations—to listen, nourish, and respond.

With pink salt, you're not just sprinkling flavor. You're reclaiming

mineral wisdom that your body has been craving all along.

Targeted Salt Rituals
by Symptom & Goal

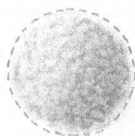

	For Belly Bloat	Salt + Digestive Spice Blends
	For Low Energy	Pink Salt + Vitamin C Combos
	For Sugar Cravings	Electrolyte Fix Tonics
	For PMS or Menopause	Magnesium + Salt Elixirs
	For Water Retention	Diuretic Herb + Salt Pairings
	For Mood Swings	Adaptogen + Salt Calming Brews

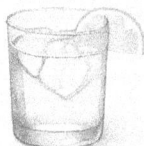

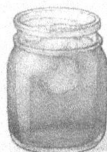

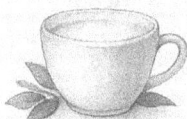

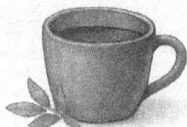

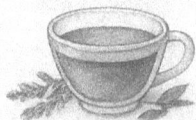

Chapter 10

Long-Term Glow — Staying Light, Balanced & Energized

What if the real secret to long-term weight loss and radiant energy wasn't harder work—but gentler rhythm?

This chapter is your invitation into that rhythm. After weeks of salt rituals, hydration resets, and metabolic balance, your body has changed. But so has your *relationship* with your body. You've learned to listen instead of punish, nourish instead of restrict. This is not the end of a plan. It's the beginning of your freedom.

Let's make it last.

1. How to Reintroduce Favorite Foods Without

Rebounding

When women experience results—less bloating, clearer skin, lifted moods—they often ask: "Can I go back to eating what I love?"

The answer is: *yes... but differently.*

The old way of reintroducing foods sounds like:

- "I've earned this," followed by a sugar binge.

- "I'm finally thin—now I can go back to 'normal.'"

- "Let me test this food, then punish myself if it causes bloat."

The new way? *Mindful re-entry.*

The Gentle Reentry Method

1. **Wait 72 Hours Between New Foods:** This gives your body space to respond and reveal any inflammation or fatigue.

2. **Watch for Subtle Clues:** Is your stomach noisier than usual? Are you sleeping more poorly? Are cravings spiking again?

3. **Don't Label Foods "Good" or "Bad":** Instead, track how foods *make you feel*. Use a simple journal (outlined below) to reflect on your energy, digestion, mood, and cycle.

4. **Prioritize Quality Over Quantity:** A homemade slice of sourdough bread with avocado is not the same as three store-bought pastries. You don't need to fear carbs—you need to upgrade their source.

5. **Support with Salt:** When reintroducing heavier meals, pair with a pink salt digestive shot (like lemon + salt water or fennel + salt blend) to reduce bloat and support bile flow.

This approach honors your metabolism, your progress, and your pleasure.

2. Creating Your Personalized Salt Ritual Journal

You've learned daily rituals, recipes, and salt combinations. But no book can teach *your body* better than *your body*.

That's why this next step matters: a simple journal that evolves with your needs.

What to Track

- **Morning Check-In**

  How did I sleep? Am I bloated, tense, or energized? What's my mood?

- **Midday Mood/Craving Log**

  Did I feel the urge to snack? What triggered it—fatigue, stress, boredom, dehydration?

- **Cycle Phase (if applicable)**

  Where am I in my hormonal rhythm? Am I in need of magnesium, warming foods, or extra rest?

- **Salt Rituals Used**

  Which ones did I do today? Did I feel better after?

- **Daily Insight (1 line only)**

  "I felt calm after my evening tonic."

  "Skipping salt made me snack more."

  "I had more energy today with lemon salt water."

Tip: Keep it on your kitchen counter or nightstand. Don't overthink—just reflect.

This journal becomes your blueprint. Over time, patterns emerge, showing you how to tweak your rituals *before* your body crashes.

3. Weekly Self-Checks: Bloat, Stress, Cycle, Sleep

Each week, carve out 10 minutes on a Sunday to gently reflect. Ask:

- **Am I holding extra water weight?**

  → Time to boost diuretic herbs or simplify evening meals.

- **Am I feeling wired, anxious, or fatigued?**

  → Consider adrenal tonics (salt + ashwagandha) or grounding baths.

- **Where am I in my menstrual or hormonal cycle?**

  → PMS phase? Add magnesium + salt. Ovulation? Increase hydration.

- **How's my sleep quality?**

  → Struggling? Try an earlier dinner, less screen time, and a salt-lavender infusion.

The goal is not perfection. It's awareness. From that space, you can adjust your rhythm without judgment.

4. Morning vs. Evening Salt Rituals Based on Your Energy Type

Your energy has a pattern. Learning it is a superpower.

If You're a Morning Slow-Starter...

- **Morning:** Warm salt-lemon water + light movement

- **Midday:** Salted green smoothie or energizing broth

- **Evening:** Magnesium-salt calm tonic to prevent night-time restlessness

If You're a Night Owl or Overthinker...

- **Morning:** Light ginger-salt infusion to gently wake the body

- **Midday:** Salt + adaptogen tea (like rhodiola or holy basil)

- **Evening:** Salt-lavender or fennel-salt drink to slow your mind

If You Crash Midday...

- **Morning:** Salted tonic with vitamin C-rich fruits (grapefruit or orange)

- **Midday:** Himalayan salt + coconut water

- **Evening:** Salt + lemon balm drink

These are not "rules," just rhythms. Test. Observe. Adjust. No two women respond exactly the same—and that's the beauty of it.

5. The New Wellness: Balance, Not Restriction

What if *lightness* was no longer about subtraction?

Not about eating less. But about *carrying less*—less shame, less fear, less perfectionism.

The Pink Salt Trick was never about avoiding food. It was about *remembering how to nourish your body's core needs: minerals, rhythm, and breath.*

What Balance Looks Like Long-Term

- You eat the cake and know how to recover with salt tonic the next day
- You skip a ritual, and instead of guilt, you give yourself extra water and love

168

- You wake up bloated, but you *know what to do*—you're no longer confused or desperate

This is a shift from *control* to *connection*. That's real wellness.

6. Staying Consistent Through Mindset Shifts — Not Willpower

Willpower is a trap. It says, "You have to fight yourself."

But mindset—the kind that lasts—says: "You're on the same team as your body."

Here's how to build that:

Ritual, Not Routine

Routine is robotic. Ritual is sacred.

Make your salt tea in a quiet moment, light a candle, play soft music.

Let it become an act of devotion.

Self-Compassion Over Self-Critique

You *will* have days you forget. That's not failure—it's feedback.

Notice. Reflect. Reset.

Identity, Not Motivation

Instead of saying "I have to keep going," say:

"This is who I am now. A woman who listens to her body."

That single identity shift rewires every decision.

Final Reflection

Staying light and energized isn't about always doing things right.

It's about knowing what brings you back home to yourself.

You now have the tools:

Salt to support your rhythms

Journaling to decode your body's signals

Mindset shifts that build consistency with *grace* instead of force

Let this chapter be the doorway—not the end—of your new life.

You don't need another diet.

You need your own daily rhythm.

And now… you have it.

Long-Term Glow —
Staying Light, Balanced & Energized

How to reintroduce favorite foods without rebounding

☑ energy
☑ digestion
☑ mood
☐ cycle

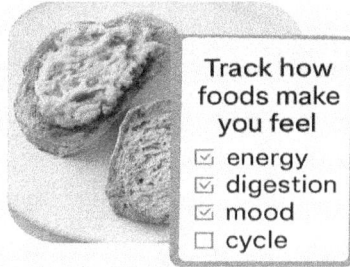

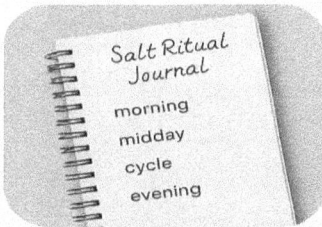

Track how foods make you feel

☑ energy
☑ digestion
☑ mood
☐ cycle

Salt Ritual Journal

morning
midday
cycle
evening

Creating your personalized salt ritual journal

Weekly self–checks: bloat, stress, cycle, sleep

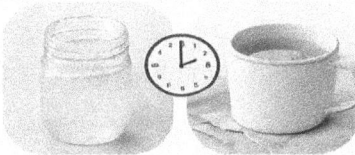

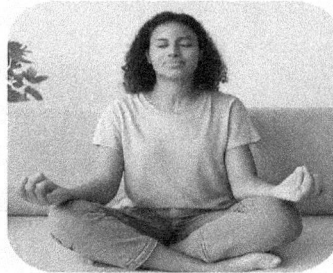

Weekly self-checks: bloat, stress, cycle, sleep

The new approach to wellness: balance, not restriction
Staying consistent through mindset shifts, not

Chapter 11

You Don't Need to Diet to Change Your Life

There comes a moment in every woman's wellness journey when she realizes that the problem was never her body. It was the noise. The guilt. The punishment disguised as willpower. The shame dressed up as discipline. The culture that taught us that being light, beautiful, or worthy meant being small, hungry, and tired.

But not anymore.

This book was never about another rule. It's not another silent war against your reflection. It's a return. A remembering. A coming home to the body you live in — not as something to fix or fight — but as something to support, nourish, and partner with.

Letting Go of Control, Guilt & Punishment

If you've made it here, something in you already knows the truth: control doesn't equal freedom. Guilt doesn't equal growth. And punishment doesn't equal change.

The real work — the deep, lasting transformation — doesn't come from tracking calories, counting macros, or berating yourself for not being "disciplined enough." It comes from trusting your body again. From listening to the whispers before they become screams. From giving your body the minerals, water, breath, rhythm, and rest it's been quietly asking for all along.

This is not about never eating chocolate again. It's about no longer needing it to feel safe. It's not about eliminating carbs. It's about eliminating the fear that makes you binge. It's not about eating "clean." It's about living clean — in your thoughts, your rituals, your relationship with your needs.

You don't have to earn the right to feel good. You just have to stop standing in your own way.

Embracing Rituals Over Rules

If diets are prisons, then rituals are the keys that set us free.

A ritual isn't a punishment. It's a gift. It's a message to your nervous system that says, "You're safe now. I've got you." Whether it's your morning pink salt tonic, your bedtime salt-magnesium soak, or your journaling moment between bites — these small acts are more than habits. They are anchors.

They anchor you in presence. In intention. In care.

Unlike diets, rituals don't demand perfection. They don't shame you when life gets messy. They meet you where you are — with open arms — and say, "Let's try again."

Rituals are sustainable because they're soulful. They become second nature. And as you've seen throughout this book, salt — simple, humble, mineral-rich — is one of the most powerful tools to root those rituals in real physiological change.

Every time you stir it into your drink, every time you taste it on your food, every time you sip your tea or massage your skin or ground your breath — you are reminding your body that healing is possible. That nourishment is available. That wellness isn't a fight — it's a flow.

Becoming the Calm, Light & Energized Version of You

You may not see it all at once. But you'll feel it.

- You'll wake up with clearer energy and a lighter body.
- You'll crave less and feel more satisfied.
- Your sleep will deepen.

- Your mind will soften.

- Your mood will lift.

- You'll notice your skin glowing, your belly less puffy, your clothes fitting differently — not because you punished your body into change, but because you partnered with it.

This is the version of you that doesn't chase trends — she honors her cycles.

This is the version of you that doesn't panic when plans change — she listens inward and adjusts with grace.

This is the version of you who chooses softness over severity, nourishment over numbers, and consistency over chaos.

You are not broken. You were just taught the wrong tools.

And now you have better ones.

You have the pink salt ritual. You have recipes, plans, and reminders that healing doesn't have to hurt. You've seen what's possible — not just in your weight, but in your wholeness.

So take a deep breath, dear reader. You made it.

You're not starting another diet. You're ending the war.

Welcome to the rest of your life — the lighter, freer, better-fed one.

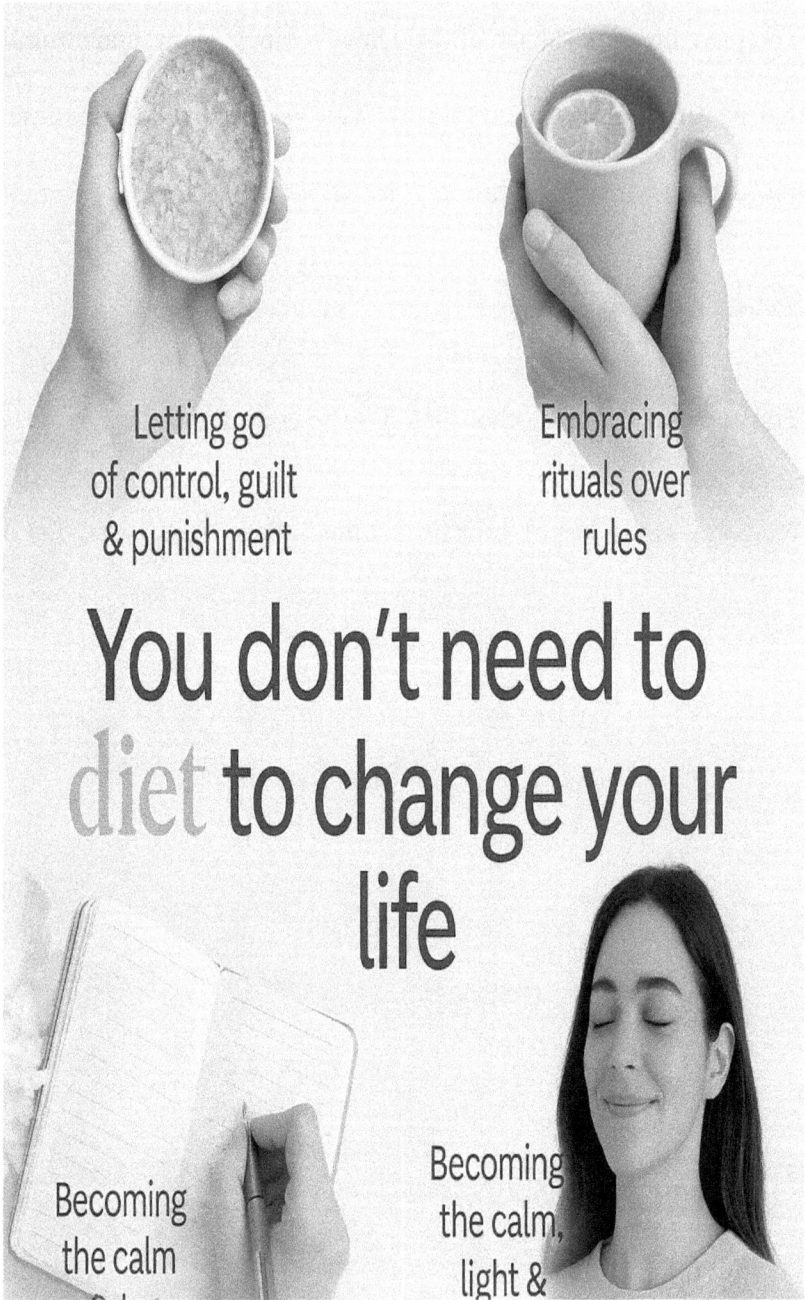

Letting go
of control, guilt
& punishment

Embracing
rituals over
rules

You don't need to diet to change your life

Becoming
the calm

Becoming
the calm,
light &

Acknowledgments

To the quiet mornings and the healing rituals that whispered, "Start here."

To every woman who ever felt bloated, tired, confused, or defeated by her own body—I wrote this for you.

Thank you to my readers, friends, and early testers who believed in the power of pink salt before the world caught on. Your stories, feedback, and transformations gave this book its heartbeat.

www.ingramcontent.com/pod-product-compliance
Lightning Source LLC
Chambersburg PA
CBHW031125020426
42333CB00012B/240